Azicip-500

Scott Horrell

Azithromycin

Azithromycin is utilized to treat specific bacterial contaminations, like bronchitis; pneumonia; physically communicated illnesses (sexually transmitted disease); and contaminations of the ears, lungs, sinuses, skin, throat, and conceptive organs. Azithromycin additionally is utilized to treat or forestall spread Mycobacterium avium complex (Macintosh) contamination [a kind of lung disease that frequently influences individuals with human immunodeficiency infection (HIV)]. Azithromycin is in a class of prescriptions called macrolide anti-toxins. It works by halting the development of microscopic organisms.

Anti-infection agents, for example, azithromycin won't work for colds, influenza, or other viral diseases. Utilizing anti-toxins when they are not required expands your gamble of getting a contamination later that opposes anti-infection treatment.

Azithromycin comes as a tablet, a drawn out discharge (long-acting) suspension (fluid), and a suspension (fluid) to take by mouth. The tablets and suspension (Zithromax) are typically taken regardless of food once every day for 1-5 days. When utilized for the counteraction of scattered Macintosh disease, azithromycin tablets are normally taken regardless of food once week after week. The lengthy delivery suspension (Zmax) is generally taken while starving (something like 1 hour prior or 2 hours after a dinner) as a one-time portion. To assist you with making sure to take azithromycin, take it around a similar time consistently. Follow the headings on your medicine mark cautiously, and ask you're PCP or drug specialist to make sense of any part you don't have any idea. Take azithromycin precisely as coordinated. Try not to take pretty much of it or take it more frequently than endorsed by your PCP.

Shake the fluid well before each utilization to equally blend the drug. Utilize a dosing spoon, oral needle, or estimating cup to gauge the right measure of prescription. Flush the estimating gadget with water subsequent to taking the full portion of medicine.

Assuming you get azithromycin powder for suspension (Zithromax) in the single-portion, 1-gram bundle, you should initially blend it in with water before you take the prescription. Blend the items in the 1-gram bundle with 1/4 cup (60 mL) of water in a glass and drink the whole items right away. Add an extra 1/4 cup (60 mL) of water to a similar glass, blend, and drink the whole items to guarantee that you get the whole portion.

In the event that you get azithromycin expanded discharge suspension (Zmax) as a dry powder, you should initially add water to the container before you take the drug. Open the container by pushing down on the cap and bending. Measure 1/4 cup (60 mL) of water, and add to the jug. Close the jug firmly, and shake well to blend. Utilize the azithromycin broadened discharge suspension in no less than 12 hours of getting it from the drug store or in the wake of adding water to the powder.

Assuming that you upchuck soon after taking azithromycin, summon your PCP right. Your primary care physician will let you know if you really want to take another portion. Try not to take another portion except if your PCP advises you to do as such.

You ought to start to feel improved during the initial not many long stretches of treatment with azithromycin. On the off chance that your side effects don't improve, or deteriorate, call your primary care physician.

Take azithromycin until you finish the solution, regardless of whether you feel improved. Try not to quit taking azithromycin except if you experience the extreme aftereffects depicted in the Secondary effects segment. On the off chance that you quit taking azithromycin too early or skip portions, your contamination may not be totally treated and the microbes might become impervious to anti-infection agents.

Prior to taking azithromycin,

let your primary care physician and drug specialist know if you are hypersensitive to azithromycin, clarithromycin (Biaxin, in Prevpac), dirithromycin (not accessible in the U.S.), erythromycin (E.E.S., ERYC, Erythrocin), telithromycin (Ketek; not accessible in the U.S.), some other prescriptions, or any of the fixings in azithromycin tablets or suspension (fluid). Request your drug specialist for a rundown from the fixings.

tell your primary care physician and drug specialist what other medicine and nonprescription prescriptions, nutrients, nourishing enhancements, and natural items you are taking or plan to take. Make certain to specify any of the accompanying: anticoagulants ('blood thinners') like warfarin for incidental effects.

in the event that you are taking acid neutralizers containing aluminum hydroxide or magnesium hydroxide (Maalox, Mylanta, Tums, others), you should permit a chance to pass between when you take a portion of these acid neutralizers and when you take a portion of azithromycin tablets or fluid. Ask your PCP or drug specialist what amount of time previously or after you require for azithromycin you might take these meds. The lengthy delivery suspension might be taken out of the blue with acid neutralizers.

Let your primary care physician know if you have at any point had jaundice (yellowing of the skin or eyes) or other liver issues while taking azithromycin. Your primary care physician will likely tell you not to take azithromycin.

let your primary care physician know if you or anybody in your family has or has at any point had a delayed QT stretch (an uncommon heart issue that might cause sporadic heartbeat, swooning, or unexpected demise) or a quick, slow, or unpredictable heartbeat, and assuming that you have low degrees of magnesium or potassium in your blood; assuming you have a blood contamination; cardiovascular breakdown or other heart issues; cystic fibrosis; myasthenia gravis (a state of muscles and the nerves that control them); or then again on the off chance that you have kidney or liver sickness.

Let your PCP know if you are pregnant, plan to become pregnant, or are breastfeeding. Assuming you becomes pregnant while taking azithromycin, call your PCP.

Azithromycin might cause secondary effects. Let your primary care physician knows if any of these side effects are serious or don't disappear:

Sickness

Loose bowels

Heaving

Stomach torment

Cerebral pain

A few incidental effects can be serious. Assuming that you experience any of these side effects, quit accepting azithromycin and call your primary care physician right away or seek crisis clinical treatment:

Quick, beating, or sporadic heartbeat

Tipsiness

Blacking out

Rash regardless of a fever

Rankles or stripping

Fever and discharge filled; rankle like injuries, redness, and enlarging of the skin

Hives

Tingling

Wheezing or trouble breathing or gulping

Expanding of the face, throat, tongue, lips, eyes, hands, feet, lower legs, or lower legs

Dryness

Retching or peevishness while taking care of (in newborn children under about a month and a half old)

Serious loose bowels (watery or horrendous stools) that might happen regardless of fever and stomach cramps (may happen as long as 2 months or more after your treatment)

Yellowing of the skin or eyes

Outrageous sleepiness

Strange draining or swelling

Absence of energy

Loss of craving

Torment in the upper right piece of the stomach

Influenza like side effects

Dull hued pee

Surprising muscle shortcoming or trouble with muscle control

Pink and enlarged eyes

Features for azithromycin

Azithromycin oral tablet is accessible as both a conventional and brand-name drug. Brand name: Zithromax.

Azithromycin comes as a tablet and suspension, the two of which are taken by mouth. It likewise comes as eye drops, as well as an intravenous structure that is given by a medical services supplier.

Azithromycin is utilized to treat contaminations brought about by specific microorganisms.

Significant admonitions

Unusual heart mood cautioning. In certain individuals, azithromycin might cause a strange heart beat called QT prolongation. The gamble of this condition is expanded assuming you as of now dislike your heart mood or on the other hand on the off chance that you consume different medications that may likewise cause QT prolongation. The gamble is additionally expanded in more seasoned grown-ups. QT prolongation is intense, and it might try and be deadly at times. On the off chance that you dislike your heart cadence, tell your primary care physician prior to taking azithromycin. Additionally enlighten your primary care physician concerning any remaining meds you're taking prior to beginning this medication.

Anti-microbial related loose bowels cautioning. Practically all anti-toxins, including azithromycin, can cause the runs. The medication might make gentle loose bowels serious irritation of your colon, which can cause demise. Call your PCP assuming you have serious looseness of the bowels or the runs that endure after you quit taking this medication.

Liver issues cautioning. In uncommon cases, this medication can lead to liver issues. Assuming you as of now have liver sickness, it could deteriorate your liver capability. During treatment with azithromycin, your primary care physician might have to screen your liver capability. They might do blood tests to check how well your liver is functioning. On the off chance that your liver isn't functioning admirably, your PCP might have you quit taking this medication.

Myasthenia gravis cautioning. Azithromycin can deteriorate side effects of myasthenia gravis, a condition that causes side effects, for example, shortcoming in muscles utilized for development.

Azithromycin can likewise cause a comparative condition called myasthenic disorder. Assuming that you have myasthenia gravis, make certain to tell your primary care physician prior to taking azithromycin.

Macrolide, class of anti-infection agents described by their huge lactone ring structures and by their development hindering (bacteriostatic) impacts on microorganisms. The macrolides were first found during the 1950s, when researchers disconnected erythromycin from the dirt bacterium Streptomyces erythraeus. During the 1970s and 1980s manufactured subsidiaries of erythromycin, including clarithromycin and azithromycin, were created.

Macrolides are generally managed orally; however they can be given parenterally. These medications are important in treating pharyngitis and pneumonia brought about by Streptococcus in people delicate to penicillin. They are utilized in treating pneumonias caused either by Mycoplasma species or by Legionella pneumophila (the creature that causes Legionnaire illness); they are additionally utilized in treating pharyngeal transporters of Corynebacterium diphtheriae, the bacillus liable for diphtheria.

Macrolides work by restricting to a particular subunit of ribosomes (destinations of protein union) in helpless microorganisms, in this way hindering the development of bacterial proteins. In many living beings this activity represses cell development; in any case, in high focuses it can cause cell demise. A few types of microscopic organisms, including Streptococcus pneumoniae and Staphylococcus aureus, have been found to convey changes that modify the macrolide restricting site on the ribosomal subunit, which delivers the microorganisms impervious to the specialists. Different systems of protection from macrolides, including the enactment of medication efflux proteins and the creation of medication inactivating compounds, likewise have arisen in certain kinds of microscopic organisms.

Minor results of macrolides incorporate sickness, spewing, the runs, and ringing or humming in the ears (tinnitus). Serious aftereffects, including hypersensitive response and cholestatic hepatitis (irritation and clog of bile conduits in the liver), are for the most part related exclusively with the utilization of erythromycin. Macrolides likewise have significant medication cooperations that can prompt unfriendly effects on the heart.

Antibiotic medication, any of a gathering of expansive range anti-infection intensifies that have a typical essential design and are either disconnected straightforwardly from a few types of Streptomyces microorganisms or created semi synthetically from those segregated mixtures.

Antibiotic medications act by obstructing the capacity of a bacterium to deliver specific essential proteins; in this manner, they are inhibitors of development (bacteriostatic) as opposed to enemies of the irresistible specialist (bacteriocidal) and are viable just against duplicating microorganisms. Antibiotic medications are utilized against different irresistible illnesses, including cholera, rickettsial contaminations, trachoma (a constant contamination of the eye), psittacosis (a sickness sent by specific birds), brucellosis, and tularemia. Antibiotic medications have likewise been utilized for the treatment of skin inflammation.

While all antibiotic medications have a typical design, they contrast from one another by the presence or nonappearance of chloride, methyl, and hydroxyl gatherings. Albeit these alterations don't change their expansive range antibacterial movement, they really do influence pharmacological properties like half-life and restricting to proteins in serum. The antibiotic medications all have a similar antibacterial range, despite the fact that there are distinctions in responsiveness of the microbes to the different kinds of antibiotic medications. They restrain protein amalgamation in both bacterial and human cells. Microscopic organisms have a framework that permits antibiotic medications to be moved into the cell, while human cells don't; human cells hence are saved the impacts of antibiotic medication on protein blend.

All antibiotic medications are consumed from the gastrointestinal parcel after oral organization, and most can be given intravenously or intramuscularly. Since calcium, magnesium, aluminum, and iron structure insoluble items with most antibiotic medications, they can't be given at the same time with substances containing these minerals (e.g., milk). Buildings among antibiotic medications and calcium can cause staining of teeth and hindrance of bone development in small kids or in babies assuming antibiotic medications are required after the fourth month of pregnancy. Antibiotic medication can likewise cause photosensitivity in patients presented to daylight.

Since not the antibiotic medication regulated orally is all retained from the gastrointestinal lot, the bacterial populace of the digestive tract can become impervious to antibiotic medications, bringing about abundance (suprainfection) of safe organic entities. The far reaching utilization of antibiotic medications is remembered to have added to an expansion in the quantity of antibiotic medication safe life forms, thusly delivering specific contaminations stronger to treatment. The utilization of antibiotic medications in domesticated animals feed to advance development has additionally been raised doubt about.

Anti-toxin, synthetic substance delivered by a living life form, for the most part a microorganism that is negative to different microorganisms. Anti-toxins regularly are created by soil microorganisms and presumably address a method by which organic entities in a complicated climate, for example, soil, control the development of contending microorganisms. Microorganisms that produce anti-microbials valuable in forestalling or treating illness incorporate the microbes and the parasites.

Anti-microbials came into overall unmistakable quality with the presentation of penicillin in 1941. From that point forward they have changed the treatment of bacterial diseases in people and different creatures. They are, be that as it may, insufficient against infections.

The principal anti-toxins

In 1928 Scottish bacteriologist Alexander Fleming saw that states of microorganisms developing on a culture plate had been negatively impacted by a form, Penicillium notatum, which had debased the way of life. After 10 years English organic chemist Ernst Chain, Australian pathologist Howard Florey, and others segregated the fixing mindful, penicillin, and showed that it was exceptionally successful against numerous serious bacterial contaminations. Close to the furthest limit of the 1950s researchers explored different avenues regarding the expansion of different synthetic gatherings to the center of the penicillin atom to produce semisynthetic variants. A scope of penicillins in this way opened up to treat illnesses brought about by various kinds of microbes, including staphylococci, streptococci, pneumococci, gonococci, and the spirochaetes of syphilis.

Obviously unaffected by penicillin was the tubercle bacillus (Mycobacterium tuberculosis). This creature, nonetheless, ended up being profoundly delicate to streptomycin, an anti-toxin that was detached from Streptomyces griseus in 1943. As well as being decisively viable against tuberculosis, streptomycin showed movement against numerous different sorts of microbes, including the typhoid fever bacillus. Two other early disclosures were gramicidin and tyrocidin, which are created by microbes of the class Bacillus. Found in 1939 by French-conceived American microbiologist René Dubos, they were significant in treating shallow diseases yet were excessively poisonous for inward use.

During the 1950s specialists found the cephalosporins, which are connected with penicillins however are delivered by the form Cephalosporium acrimonious. The next decade researchers found a class of anti-toxins known as quinolones. Quinolones intrude on the replication of DNA — a vital stage in bacterial propagation — and have demonstrated valuable in treating urinary parcel diseases, irresistible looseness of the bowels, and different contaminations including components like bones and white platelets.

Use and organization of anti-infection agents

The rule overseeing the utilization of anti-infection agents is to guarantee that the patient gets one to which the objective bacterium is delicate, at a sufficiently high fixation to be powerful yet not cause secondary effects, and for an adequate period of time to guarantee that the disease is completely killed. Anti-infection agents shift in their scope of activity. Some are profoundly unambiguous. Others, like the antibiotic medications, act against a wide range of various microscopic organisms. These are especially valuable in battling blended diseases and in treating contaminations when there is no chance to lead responsiveness tests. While certain anti-microbials, like the semisynthetic penicillins and the quinolones, can be taken orally, others should be given by intramuscular or intravenous infusion.

Systems of activity

Anti-microbials produce their results through different components of activity. A huge number work by repressing bacterial cell wall combination; these specialists are alluded to for the most part as β-lactam anti-microbials. Creation of the bacterial cell wall includes the fractional gathering of wall parts inside the phone, transport of these designs through the phone film to the developing wall, get together into the wall, lastly cross-connecting of the strands of wall material. Anti-microbials that restrain the union of the cell wall explicitly affect some stage. The outcomes are a change in the cell wall and state of the creature and at last the passing of the bacterium.

Different anti-infection agents, for example, the aminoglycosides, chloramphenicol, erythromycin, and clindamycin, repress protein blend in microscopic organisms. The essential interaction by which microbes and creature cells orchestrate proteins is comparative, yet the proteins included are unique. Those anti-infection agents that are specifically poisonous use these distinctions to tie to or repress the capability of the proteins of the bacterium, subsequently forestalling the union of new proteins and new bacterial cells.

Anti-toxins like polymyxin B and polymyxin E (colistin) tie to phospholipids in the cell layer of the bacterium and disrupt its capability as a specific hindrance; this permits fundamental macromolecules in the cell to spill out, bringing about the demise of the phone. Since different cells, including human cells, have comparable or indistinguishable phospholipids, these anti-infection agents are to some degree poisonous.

A few anti-infection agents, like the sulfonamides, are cutthroat inhibitors of the union of folic corrosive (folate), which is a fundamental primer move toward the combination of nucleic acids. Sulfonamides can hinder folic corrosive amalgamation since they are like a transitional compound (para-aminobenzoic corrosive) that is switched by a chemical over completely to folic corrosive. The similitude in structure between these mixtures brings about rivalry between para-aminobenzoic corrosive and the sulfonamide for the protein answerable for switching the middle of the road over completely to folic corrosive. This response is reversible by eliminating the compound, which brings about the restraint yet not the demise of the microorganisms. One anti-microbial, rifampin disrupts ribonucleic corrosive (RNA) blend in microscopic organisms by restricting to a subunit on the bacterial chemical liable for duplication of RNA. Since the proclivity of rifampin is a lot more grounded for the bacterial protein than for the human catalyst, the human cells are unaffected at remedial dosages.

Anti-microbial opposition

An issue that has tormented anti-infection treatment from the earliest days is the obstruction that microorganisms can create to the medications. An anti-microbial may kill essentially every one of the microorganisms causing an illness in a patient, however a couple of microscopic organisms that are hereditarily less helpless against the impacts of the medication might make due. These proceed to imitate or to move their protection from others of their species through cycles of quality trade. With their more weak rivals cleared out or diminished in numbers by anti-microbials, these safe strains multiply. The outcome is bacterial diseases in people that are untreatable by one or even a few of the anti-infection agents generally compelling in such cases. The unpredictable and inaccurate utilization of anti-toxins empowers the spread of such bacterial opposition. (See anti-infection opposition.)

Specialists are ceaselessly attempting to find new anti-microbials for the purpose of conquering anti-toxin obstruction. A few possibly successful mixtures that have been found incorporate specific bacterial poisons and antimicrobial peptides. Novel treatment procedures, like consolidating synergistic anti-toxins to help the killing of microbes, are additionally being scrutinized. It could be feasible to bring compounds into bacterial populaces that really desensitize the microscopic organisms to existing anti-toxin drugs.

Each kind of anti-microbial has a particular application in medication and can act as a helpful model for investigating the different systems by which anti-toxins apply their belongings. The accompanying segments center around the penicillins and cephalosporins, imipenem, the antituberculosis anti-microbials, and the specialists aztreonam, bacitracin, and vancomycin. These specialists and gatherings of specialists further show the substance and practical variety found among the anti-toxins.

The penicillins have an exceptional construction, a β-lactam ring that is liable for their antibacterial movement. The β-lactam ring connects with proteins in the bacterial cell liable for the last move toward the get together of the phone wall.

The penicillins can be isolated into two gatherings: the normally happening penicillins (penicillin G, penicillin V, and benzathine penicillin) and the semisynthetic penicillins. The semisynthetic penicillins are created by developing the shape Penicillium under conditions by which just the essential atom (6-aminopenicillanic corrosive) is delivered. By adding specific compound gatherings to this particle, a few different semisynthetic penicillins are delivered that change in protection from corruption by β-lactamase (penicillinase), a catalyst that explicitly breaks the β-lactam ring, consequently inactivating the anti-infection. Furthermore, the antibacterial range of action and pharmacological properties of the regular penicillins can be changed and worked on by these substance alterations. The expansion of a β-lactamase inhibitor, for example, clavulanic corrosive, to penicillin decisively works on the viability of the anti-toxin. A few normally happening inhibitors have been confined, and others have been synthetically blended.

The normally happening penicillins stay the medications of decision for treating streptococcal sore throat, tonsillitis, endocarditis brought about by certain streptococci, syphilis, and meningococcal contaminations. A few microbes, most eminently Staphylococcus, created protection from the normally happening penicillins, which prompted the development of the penicillinase-safe penicillins (methicillin, oxacillin, nafcillin, cloxacillin, and dicloxacillin). The utilization of a few of these specialists, be that as it may, has been seriously restricted by obstruction; methicillin is not generally utilized, in view of the rise of methicillin-safe Staphylococcus aureus (MRSA).

To expand the value of the penicillins to the treatment of diseases brought about by gram-negative bars, the wide range penicillins (ampicillin, amoxicillin, carbenicillin, and ticarcillin) were created. These penicillins are delicate to penicillinase, yet they are valuable in treating urinary lot contaminations brought about by gram-negative bars as well as in treating typhoid and intestinal fevers.

The lengthy range specialists (mezlocillin and piperacillin) are remarkable in that they have more noteworthy movement against gram-pessimistic microbes, including Pseudomonas aeruginosa, a bacterium that frequently causes serious contamination in individuals whose resistant frameworks have been debilitated. They have diminished action, notwithstanding, against penicillinase-delivering Staphylococcus aureus, a typical bacterial specialist in food contamination.

The penicillins are the most secure of all anti-microbials. The major unfriendly response related with their utilization is excessive touchiness, with responses going from a rash to bronchospasm and hypersensitivity. The more serious responses are extraordinary.

Cephalosporins

The cephalosporins have a system of activity indistinguishable from that of the penicillins. Be that as it may, the essential substance construction of the penicillins and cephalosporins varies in different regards, bringing about some distinction in the range of antibacterial action. Change of the essential atom (7-aminocephalosporanic corrosive) created by Cephalosporium acremonium brought about four ages of cephalosporins. The original cephalosporins (cefazolin, cephalothin, and cephalexin) have a scope of antibacterial action like the expansive range penicillins portrayed previously. For example, they are viable against most staphylococci and streptococci as well as penicillin-safe pneumococci.

The second-age cephalosporins (cefamandole, cefaclor, cefotetan, cefoxitin, and cefuroxime) have a lengthy antibacterial range that incorporates more noteworthy movement against extra types of gram-negative bars. Hence, these medications are dynamic against Escherichia coli and Klebsiella and Proteus species (however a few types of these creatures have created obstruction). Cefamandole is dynamic against many types of Haemophilus influenzae and Enterobacter, while cefoxitin is especially dynamic against most kinds of Bacteroides fragilis. Second-age cephalosporins have diminished action, be that as it may, against gram-positive microscopic organisms.

The third-age cephalosporins (ceftriaxone, cefixime, and ceftazidime) have expanded movement against the gram-negative living beings contrasted and the second-age specialists. Most Enterobacter species are vulnerable to these medications, as are H. influenzae and different types of Neisseria. The antibacterial range of the fourth-age compounds (cefepime) is like that of the third-age drugs, yet the fourth-age drugs. The third-age cephalosporins (ceftriaxone, cefixime, and ceftazidime) have expanded action against the gram-negative life forms contrasted and the second-age specialists. Most Enterobacter species are defenseless to these medications, as are H. influenzae and different types of Neisseria. The antibacterial range of the fourth-age compounds (cefepime) is like that of the third-age drugs, yet the fourth-age drugs have more protection from β-lactamases.

Like the penicillins, the cephalosporins are generally nontoxic. Since the design of the cephalosporins is like that of penicillin, extreme touchiness responses can happen in penicillin-easily affected patients.

Imipenem

Imipenem is a β-lactam anti-microbial that works by disrupting cell wall blend. It is profoundly impervious to hydrolysis by most β-lactamases. This medication should be given by intramuscular infusion or intravenous mixture since it isn't ingested from the gastrointestinal parcel. Imipenem is hydrolyzed by a catalyst present in the renal tubule; consequently, it is constantly managed with cilastatin, an inhibitor of this protein. Neurotoxicity and seizures have restricted the utilization of imipenem.

Antituberculosis anti-toxins

Isoniazid, ethambutol, pyrazinamide, and ethionamide are engineered synthetics utilized in treating tuberculosis. Isoniazid, ethionamide, and pyrazinamide are comparative in construction to nicotinamide adenine dinucleotide (NAD), a coenzyme fundamental for a few physiological cycles. Ethambutol forestalls the combination of mycolic corrosive, a lipid found in the tubercule bacillus. This multitude of medications is ingested from the gastrointestinal plot and infiltrate tissues and cells. An isoniazid-actuated hepatitis can happen, especially in patients 35 years old or more seasoned. Cycloserine, an anti-microbial delivered by Streptomyces orchidaceus, is additionally utilized in the treatment of tuberculosis. An underlying simple of the amino corrosive D-alanine, it impedes catalysts essential for fuse of D-alanine into the bacterial cell wall. It is quickly consumed from the gastrointestinal lot and enters most tissues very well; undeniable levels are tracked down in pee. Rifampin, a semisynthetic specialist, is retained from the gastrointestinal parcel, enters tissue well (counting the lung), and is utilized in the treatment of tuberculosis. Rifampin organization is related with a few secondary effects, generally gastrointestinal in nature. The medication can turn pee, dung, spit, sweat, and tears red-orange in variety.

Aztreonam, bacitracin, and vancomycin

Aztreonam is an engineered anti-microbial that works by hindering cell wall union, and it is normally impervious to some β-lactamases. Aztreonam has a low rate of poisonousness; however it should be controlled parenterally.

Bacitracin is created by an extraordinary type of Bacillus subtilis. As a result of its serious poisonousness to kidney cells, its utilization is restricted to the skin treatment of skin diseases brought about by Streptococcus and Staphylococcus and for eye and ear contaminations.

Vancomycin, an anti-infection created by Streptomyces orientalism, is inadequately ingested from the gastrointestinal lot and is generally given by intravenous infusion. It is utilized for the treatment of serious staphylococcal diseases brought about by strains impervious to the different penicillins. Its utilization against MRSA prompted the development of vancomycin-safe Staphylococcus aureus (VRSA).

Azithromycin is an antimicrobial drug used to treat and oversee bacterial contaminations, including local area obtained pneumonia and physically sent illnesses. It is in the macrolide class of antimicrobials. The issues treated by azithromycin are significant reasons for irresistible sickness grimness and mortality in the US. This action surveys the signs, contraindications, system of activity, and poison levels of azithromycin treatment in the clinical setting and significant endorsing and the executive's contemplations for the medical services group.

Recognize the component of activity and organization of azithromycin.

Depict the unfriendly impacts and contraindications of azithromycin.

Sum up the fitting checking of azithromycin treatment and its poison levels. Audit contemplations applicable to the interprofessional group and examine procedures for improving patient results and care coordination.

Azithromycin (ay zith" roe mye' sin) is a semisynthetic macrolide anti-toxin utilized generally to treat gentle to-direct bacterial diseases brought about by delicate specialists. Azithromycin, as other macrolide anti-toxins like erythromycin and clarithromycin, is bacteriostatic against numerous gram positive microorganisms including many types of streptococci, staphylococci, clostridia, corynebacteria, listeria, haemophilus sp., moxicella, and Neisseria meningitidis. Azithromycin is more dynamic than erythromycin against a few gram negative microbes as well as Mycoplasma pneumonia, Helicobacter pylori, Toxoplasma gondii, cryptosporidium and a few abnormal mycobacteria. Macrolide anti-toxins act by repressing protein union of microbes by restricting to the 50S ribosomal component. Obstruction happens by a few instruments. Azithromycin was endorsed for use in the US in 1994 and as of now it is the most normally recommended anti-toxin in America. Ordinary signs are local area obtained pneumonia, intense intensifications of persistent bronchitis, sinusitis, pelvic incendiary sickness, urethritis and different diseases brought about by powerless microscopic organisms. Azithromycin is additionally used to treat scattered mycobacterium avium complex diseases. Azithromycin is accessible as tablets of 250 and 500 mg and as arrangements and powders for suspension conventionally and under the name Zithromax. Azithromycin is regularly given in once everyday portions for 5 to 7 days. Persistent utilization of azithromycin is utilized to treat abnormal mycobacterial contaminations and as prophylaxis against normal bacterial contaminations in exceptionally helpless people (with cystic fibrosis, ongoing granulomatous illness, or bronchiectasis). Parenteral azithromycin is commonly given in dosages of 500 mg iv every day for the initial not many long stretches of treatment in moderate-to-extreme diseases. Azithromycin is by and large very much endured; however incidental effects can incorporate sickness, stomach torment, the runs, dyspepsia, cerebral pain, tipsiness, angioedema and rash. Extreme unfriendly responses incorporate puerile pyloric stenosis, Clostridia difficile looseness of the bowels, QTc prolongation, hepatotoxicity and serious excessive touchiness responses including

Stevens Johnson disorder and poisonous epidermal necrolysis.

Like other macrolide anti-toxins, azithromycin has been connected to a low pace of intense, transient and asymptomatic rise in serum aminotransferases which happens in 1% to 2% of patients treated for brief periods, and a to some degree higher extent of patients given azithromycin long haul.

Azithromycin can likewise seldom cause clinically clear liver injury. Since azithromycin has become so generally utilized, it has likewise become one of the more normal reasons for drug instigated liver injury. The common liver injury brought about by azithromycin looks like that depicted with other macrolides and is a self-restricted, cholestatic hepatitis, emerging inside 1 to 3 weeks of beginning treatment (Case 1). It once in a while emerges after azithromycin is paused and can happen even after a short, 2 or multi day course. Run of the mill side effects are weakness, jaundice, stomach torment and pruritus. Fever and eosinophilia may likewise be available, yet immunoallergic highlights are generally not unmistakable. This type of liver injury from azithromycin is typically harmless, however in certain cases is related with delayed jaundice and diligence of liver test anomalies for a considerable length of time or more. Liver histology in these cases by and large exhibits bile conduit misfortune, which if extreme, can bring about evaporating bile pipe condition and persistent cholestatic liver disappointment, at last requiring liver transplantation. Different cases of bile pipe misfortune and delayed cholestatic hepatitis at last determination yet might be set apart by diligent serum soluble phosphatase rises of dubious clinical importance.

Azithromycin can likewise cause hepatocellular injury with side effects and jaundice. In these cases, the idleness is ordinarily short and might be 1 to 3 days just (Case 2). Serum aminotransferase levels are extraordinarily raised and basic phosphatase values are generally not as much as two times the furthest reaches of ordinary, despite the fact that they might ascend to more elevated levels with time. The hepatocellular types of liver injury from azithromycin can be serious and lead to intense liver disappointment and demise or need for crisis liver transplantation. Nonetheless, much of the time, recuperation happens inside 4 to about two months.

Azithromycin has additionally been related with serious cutaneous responses, for example, erythema multiform, drug response with eosinophilia and foundational signs (DRESS) disorder, Stevens Johnson condition (SJS) and poisonous epidermal rot (TEN). These serious cutaneous responses are frequently connected with some level of liver injury and might be joined by clinically obvious injury with jaundice, normally with a cholestatic design. Be that as it may, the extreme cutaneous responses typically eclipse the liver injury.

In cell culture, azithromycin displays some level of antiviral movement and was displayed to repress the Extreme Intense Respiratory Disorder, Covid type 2 (SARS-CoV-2), the reason for the pandemic of serious Coronavirus pneumonia that emerged in 2019 and prompted multiple million passings around the world. Considering the antiviral movement as well as mitigating activities of azithromycin, it was reused as a likely treatment of Coronavirus. Regardless of early encouraging reports, resulting randomized controlled preliminaries found that it had no advantage in one or the other anticipation of disease or improvement of the course of Coronavirus sickness. A crisis use approval conceded to azithromycin as treatment of Coronavirus in mid-2020 was subsequently removed.

Histopathology

Azithromycin hepatotoxicity is normally related histologically with a cholestatic hepatitis like what is portrayed with erythromycin incited liver injury. Dissipated bile projects are tracked down in canaliculated with humble parenchymal aggravation and putrefaction. Entry lots frequently have more articulated aggravation described by mononuclear cells and eosinophils. The cholestasis can be significant and drawn out, and azithromycin is a notable reason for disappearing bile pipe disorder. More uncommon is hepatocellular injury, an example seen most usually with reexposure, with a short idleness to beginning and biopsy taken right off the bat over injury. The minor serum aminotransferase heights that show up during treatment with azithromycin are typically harmless, asymptomatic and resolve quickly whether azithromycin is halted. The intense hepatic injury with jaundice, be that as it may, can be drawn out and inconvenient and lead to loss of intrahepatic bile pipes and evaporating bile channel condition. The injury and jaundice might emerge after azithromycin is halted, yet appearance of jaundice in somebody on azithromycin ought to prompt its brief end. Uncommon cases of intense liver disappointment and casualty from azithromycin incited liver illness have been accounted for. People with previous, fundamental persistent liver illness might be more helpless to serious results. There is probably going to be cross reactivity in hepatic injury with other macrolide anti-microbials; however this has not been legitimate.

This was an early case report of azithromycin hepatotoxicity and obviously exhibited its ordinary clinical example of sudden beginning of sickness in something like seven days of beginning the drug — and really a couple of days in the wake of halting it. The cholestatic example of liver proteins and jaundice are common (however not constant) of azithromycin hepatotoxicity. There was no notice of indications of extreme touchiness like fever, rash, arthralgias or eosinophilia, albeit the simultaneous pneumonia might have perplexed the clinical picture. Recuperation was sensibly fast, yet the harmless result might have been on the grounds that azithromycin was allowed for 3 days in particular. This patient ought to be prompted against future openness to azithromycin; however there is little data about his dangers of liver injury with other macrolide anti-infection agents (like erythromycin or clarithromycin).

Hepatocellular liver injury due to azithromycin.

A 69 year elderly person created shortcoming, anorexia, queasiness, the runs, pruritus and jaundice 4 days in the wake of beginning oral azithromycin (1000 mg at first, then, at that point, 500 mg every day) for thought intense bronchitis. She had no set of experiences of liver infection, didn't drink liquor and had no gamble factors for viral hepatitis. Her previous clinical history included hypertension, dyslipidemia, a 50 pack year history of cigarette smoking, persistent obstructive pneumonic sickness, hypothyroidism and wretchedness for which she was taking lisinopril, simvastatin, ibuprofen, loratadine, albuterol by inhaler, levothyroxine and fluoxetine. She was additionally progressively indicative from her intense aspiratory contamination. Actual assessment uncovered jaundice yet no fever, rash or organomegaly. She was dyspneic and had basilar inspiratory pops and indications of solidification. Lab tests showed bilirubin were negative. ANA was negative; however smooth muscle counter acting agent was responsive. A chest CT showed bibasilar pneumonic combinations. She was confessed to the emergency clinic, azithromycin was held and levofloxacin began. The next day she had a respiratory capture, however was effectively resustained and put on mechanical ventilation. Ultrasound of the mid-region showed no proof of biliary check in spite of the fact that there was biliary muck and gallbladder wall thickening. Over the principal seven day stretch of affirmation her serum chemicals stayed high and serum bilirubin moved to 18.5 mg/dL. Be that as it may, her pneumonic status improved, she was effectively intubated and was ultimately released on her past prescriptions without anti-infection agents and with further developing serum catalysts. At the point when found in the short term center 2 and after 5 months, her liver tests were typical.

Azithromycin is a macrolide anti-infection that is utilized in the treatment of various bacterial contaminations in grown-ups and kids. A typical solution is for the Zithromax Z-Pak. Other macrolide anti-microbials you might have known about incorporate erythromycin and Biaxin (clarithromycin).

Amoxicillin is a beta-lactam anti-microbial, connected with penicillin, which is utilized to treat various bacterial contaminations in grown-ups and kids. Amoxicillin is an exceptionally normal remedy, and Augmentin (which contains amoxicillin in addition to clavulanate to forestall opposition) is one more extremely normal medicine endorsed for different bacterial contaminations.

Are azithromycin and amoxicillin the equivalent?

The two drugs are utilized to treat bacterial contaminations in grown-ups and youngsters. Azithromycin is in the macrolide classification of anti-microbials, while amoxicillin is in the beta-lactam/penicillin class. They work in various ways and have a few distinctions, like in signs and medication cooperations.

As a rule, only either anti-toxin will be endorsed. Continuously adhere to your medical services supplier's directions on what anti-microbial to take. At times, like pneumonia or one more kind of disease where the sort of microbes isn't yet known, the medical care supplier might endorse two anti-microbials until lab work returns that shows which anti-toxin will work.

azithromycin or amoxicillin better?

While the two medications are compelling, your medical services supplier can decide whether you truly do for sure have a bacterial disease. A viral disease doesn't answer anti-toxins and can increment drug opposition. In view of the kind of contamination, and what specific microorganisms is thought or known to cause the disease, your medical care supplier can choose if one of these medications is fitting for you.

Could I at any point utilize azithromycin or amoxicillin while pregnant?

Your medical care supplier will decide the best anti-microbial to utilize assuming you are pregnant and need an anti-infection.

Azithromycin is a pregnancy class B, yet there have not been very much controlled examinations in pregnant ladies.

Amoxicillin is additionally a pregnancy class B, and like azithromycin, there have not been satisfactory investigations with pregnant ladies.

Accordingly, azithromycin or amoxicillin ought to be recommended assuming the advantages to the mother offset the dangers to the child, and under close perception of the medical care supplier. Assuming you are pregnant or wanting to become pregnant, tell your medical services supplier.

Could I at any point utilize azithromycin or amoxicillin while breastfeeding?

The endorsing data for azithromycin suggests considering the dangers versus benefits, and in the event that it is utilized in a breastfeeding lady, the child ought to be observed for the runs, spewing, or rash.

The endorsing data for amoxicillin suggests that the drug ought to be involved with alert in breastfeeding moms.

Ladies who are breastfeeding ought to counsel their supplier in regards to the most fitting anti-microbial that will be protected during breastfeeding.

Could I at any point utilize azithromycin or amoxicillin with liquor?

While the maker's data doesn't list liquor as a contraindication to or drug communication with one or the other anti-infection, it's essential to observe that liquor can keep your body from battling a contamination. Liquor can likewise make gastrointestinal (stomach) aftereffects more regrettable.

Azithromycin versus amoxicillin: Which is more grounded?

It's challenging to look at qualities in light of the fact that every prescription is in an alternate class of anti-infection agents. They have a few likenesses and a few distinctions; however we can't actually say which is more grounded. All things considered, it is critical to take a gander at what contamination is being dealt with, what microorganisms is causing the disease, some other ailments you have and any medications you take that can cooperate with azithromycin or amoxicillin. Your medical care supplier can figure out which medication is more proper for you.

Amoxicillin versus azithromycin for Coronavirus: Which is better?

Amoxicillin and azithromycin are anti-infection agents and don't treat viral contaminations like Coronavirus. You can peruse more about Coronavirus medicines on the CDC site. It means a lot to keep awake to date on your Coronavirus immunizations to assist with forestalling difficult sickness or hospitalization.

Which is better for sinus contamination, amoxicillin, or azithromycin?

A sinus disease might be brought about by an infection or by microbes (or even a growth, in uncommon cases). If your prescriber determined you to have a bacterial sinus contamination, azithromycin or amoxicillin (or Augmentin) are proper, and exceptionally normal, medicines. Your prescriber will likewise consider sensitivities and different medications you take that might connect with azithromycin or amoxicillin.

It depends in the event that your hack is coming from a bacterial or viral contamination. In the event that you have a viral disease like the normal cool, an anti-microbial won't help by any stretch of the imagination. On the off chance that your medical services supplier feels that a bacterial contamination is causing the hack, the person will pick the anti-infection that he/she feels is bound to fix the specific disease.

Physically communicated diseases (STIs), like chlamydia, syphilis, and gonorrhea, have been on the ascent from one side of the country to the other. They disproportionally influence men who engage in sexual relations with men and transsexual ladies. Left untreated, they can prompt serious medical problems, like visual impairment, cerebrum and nerve issues, and barrenness in ladies. Condoms can impede numerous STIs. In any case, condoms are not generally utilized predictably or accurately. So specialists have been investigating different choices for forestalling STIs, particularly among those at raised risk for rehashed contaminations.

Past examinations tracked down proof that the anti-toxin doxycycline, taken not long after sex, could decrease the gamble of bacterial STIs among men who have intercourse with men. This approach is called doxycycline post exposure prophylaxis, or doxy-Kick. In any case, a few specialists have been worried that preventive utilization of anti-infection agents could prompt anti-microbial obstruction. This could lessen future choices for treating STIs and other bacterial diseases.

To find out more, a group drove by researchers at the College of California, San Francisco (UCSF) and the College of Washington, Seattle, set off to gauge the security and viability of doxy-Energy. They likewise searched for proof of anti-infection opposition. Results were distributed in the New Britain Diary of Medication on April 6, 2023.

The review selected 501 grown-ups considered at high gamble for bacterial STIs, either men who engaged in sexual relations with men or transsexual ladies. All had been determined to have a bacterial STI in the previous year and revealed having intercourse without involving a condom in the previous year. They were either living with HIV or were taking or wanting to take prescription to forestall HIV disease.

Members were haphazardly allocated to get either doxy-Kick or standard consideration. Those in the doxy-Energy bunch were told to take a 200 mg doxycycline tablet as quickly as time permits in something like 72 hours after condom less sex. Members were tried for STIs like clockwork and followed for one year.

The scientists found that the doxy-Energy bunch had a 66% lower occurrence of syphilis, gonorrhea, and chlamydia contrasted with the standard-care bunch during every three-month time span. STIs were identified in around 10% of the quarterly tests managed to those in the doxy-Energy bunch, contrasted with around 30% of those in the standard-care bunch.

Gonorrhea was the most frequently analyzed STI. The frequency of gonorrhea per quarter in the doxy-Kick bunch was around 55% lower than in the standard-care bunch. Chlamydia and syphilis were each diminished by over 80% per quarter.

The specialists found that the doxy-Enthusiasm bunch had an unassumingly higher extent of doxycycline-safe Staphylococcus aureus living in the nose following a year. Also, the frequency of gonorrhea strains impervious to the anti-toxin antibiotic medication, which is in a similar anti-toxin class as doxycycline, was 38.5% in the doxy-Energy bunch contrasted with 12.5% in the gathering with standard consideration. This finding proposes doxy-Enthusiasm could be less compelling in forestalling gonorrhea with existing antibiotic medication obstruction; in any case, the quantity of accessible gonorrhea societies was low.

"It will be vital to screen the effect of doxy-Kick on antimicrobial obstruction designs after some time, and gauge this against the showed advantage of diminished STIs and related diminished anti-infection use for STI treatment in men at raised risk for repetitive STIs," says Dr. Annie Luetkemeyer of UCSF, a co-head of the review. "Given its shown viability in a few preliminaries, doxy-Energy ought to be considered as a feature of a sexual wellbeing bundle for men who have intercourse with men and transwomen in the event that they have an expanded gamble of STIs."

Anti-toxins. Anti-toxins, frequently in a solitary portion, can fix many physically sent bacterial and parasitic contaminations, including gonorrhea, syphilis, chlamydia and trichomoniasis.

When you start anti-infection treatment, completing the prescription is essential. In the event that you don't think you'll have the option to accept drug as endorsed, tell your primary care physician. A more limited, easier course of treatment might be accessible.

What's more, it's vital to keep away from sex until seven days after you've finished anti-microbial treatment and any wounds have recuperated.

Specialists likewise recommend individuals determined to have chlamydia be retested three months after treatment since there's a high opportunity of reinfection.

Antiviral medications. On the off chance that you have herpes or HIV, you'll be recommended an antiviral medication. You'll have less herpes repeats in the event that you take day to day suppressive treatment with a solution antiviral medication. In any case, giving your accomplice herpes is as yet conceivable.

Antiviral medications can hold HIV disease in line for a long time. In any case, you will in any case convey the infection and can in any case communicate it, however the gamble is lower.

The sooner you start HIV treatment, the more successful it is. Assuming that you accept your drugs as guided, it's feasible to decrease the viral burden in the blood so it can't be distinguished. By then, you won't communicate the infection to sex accomplices.

On the off chance that you've had a STI, ask your PCP how long after treatment you should be retested.

Getting retested will guarantee that the treatment worked and that you haven't been reinfected.

Assuming tests show that you have a STI, your sex accomplices — including your ongoing accomplices and some other accomplices you've had throughout recent months to one year — should be educated so they can get tried. On the off chance that they're contaminated, they can be dealt with.

Each state has various necessities, yet most states expect that specific STIs be accounted for to the neighborhood or state wellbeing office. General wellbeing offices frequently utilize prepared infection intercession experts who can assist with informing accomplices and allude individuals for treatment.

Official, private accomplice warning can assist with restricting the spread of STIs, especially for syphilis and HIV. The training additionally controls those in danger toward guiding and the right treatment. Furthermore, since you can get some STIs at least a couple of times, accomplice notice lessen your gamble of getting reinfected.

A few meds are not reasonable for individuals with specific circumstances, and here and there a medication may possibly be utilized on the off chance that additional consideration is taken. Thus, before you begin taking azithromycin it is critical that your PCP or drug specialist knows:

On the off chance that you dislike the manner in which your liver works or the manner in which your kidneys work.

On the off chance that you realize you have a surprising heartbeat.

On the off chance that you have a muscle problem called myasthenia gravis.

On the off chance that you are taking some other drugs. This incorporates any meds you are taking which are accessible to purchase without a remedy, as well as natural and corresponding meds.

In the event that you have at any point had an unfavorably susceptible response to a medication.

Step by step instructions to take azithromycin

Before you begin taking the anti-infection, read the maker's printed data flyer from inside the pack. It will give you more data about azithromycin and give a full rundown of the incidental effects which you might insight from taking it.

Take azithromycin precisely as your PCP tells you to. It is required one time each day. Contingent on the justification for why you are taking it, you may just have to take a solitary portion or you might be given a course for 3-5 days. You're PCP or drug specialist will let you know which is appropriate for you. The headings will likewise be on the name of the pack to remind you.

At the point when azithromycin is recommended for a kid, the portion will rely on the youngster's weight. Ensure you read the name cautiously so you measure out the right measure of medication. For more youthful kids, you will be given an oral dosing needle to apportion the medication - on the off chance that you are don't know how to utilize this, request that your drug specialist show you. It is smart to offer your youngster a beverage of natural product juice subsequent to taking azithromycin, as the medication can have a somewhat severe lingering flavor.

Assuming you are taking azithromycin containers, you ought to take your portions when your stomach is vacant. This implies taking them one hour before any food, or holding on until two hours a while later. Assuming you are taking tablets or fluid medication, these can be taken either previously or after food.

In the event that you neglect to take a portion, accept it when you recollect yet don't take two dosages simultaneously.

Regardless of whether you feel your disease has cleared up, continue to take the anti-infection until the course is done (except if your primary cares physician tells you in any case). This is to keep the disease from returning and being more challenging to treat.

Seeking the most from your treatment

Assuming you are likewise taking an acid neutralizer for heartburn, it can expand the time it takes for azithromycin to be consumed by your body. Along these lines, it is suggested that you don't take heartburn cures during the two hours prior or during the two hours after you take a portion of azithromycin.

Certain individuals foster thrush (redness and irritation in the mouth or vagina) in the wake of taking a course of anti-infection agents. Assuming this happens to you; talk with your primary care physician or drug specialist for guidance.

This anti-microbial may prevent the oral typhoid immunization from working. Assuming you are having any immunizations, ensure the individual treating you realizes that you are taking this medication.

Assuming you are having an activity or dental treatment, tell the individual doing the treatment that you are taking azithromycin.

Assuming you purchase any meds, check with a drug specialist that they are reasonable to take with this anti-microbial.

Assuming you actually feel unwell subsequent to finishing your tasks of the anti-infection, plan to see your PCP.

Could azithromycin at any point create some issues?

Alongside their valuable impacts, most drugs can cause undesirable incidental effects albeit not every person encounters them. The table underneath contains probably the most widely recognized ones related with azithromycin. You will find a full rundown in the producer's data handout provided with your medication. The undesirable impacts frequently work on as your body acclimates to the new medication, yet talk with your PCP or pharmaExpected results of azithromycin

Like any prescription, azithromycin can cause secondary effects. Most are by and large gentle and determine all alone. Inquire as to whether you experience any of the accompanying:

Drug communications

Azithromycin can communicate with a few meds. Advise your PCP regarding any solution or non-prescription meds you're as of now taking or start taking, including any spices or enhancements. Only a couple of the numerous drugs and enhancements the

Your ongoing utilization of all remedy and non-prescription drugs, whether every day or incidental

Any different kinds of feedback you might have about taking this medicine

The most effective method to quit taking azithromycin

You ought to keep accepting azithromycin as coordinated by your prescriber. Try not to quit taking the anti-infection except if educated to do as such, regardless of whether you're feeling much improved. Halting mid-treatment expands the gamble of fostering a repeat of your disease or an anti-microbial safe contamination.

Drug endorsement history

Azithromycin was at first found by the Croatian drug organization Pliva during the last part of the 1970s. During their underlying preliminaries, the anti-microbial substantiated it strong and equipped for staying in the body longer than different anti-toxins. However, it required a long time for the organization to profit from that discovery.[28]

In 1981, Pliva documented a patent in the nation once known as Yugoslavia, then around the world. Those underlying licenses ended up being the way in to the anti-toxin's prosperity. Pfizer researchers looking through the US Patent and Exchange Office perceived its huge potential. By 1986, Pliva and Pfizer arrived at a commonly helpful permitting understanding. Azithromycin accomplished FDA endorsement in 1991 to be sold under the brand name Zithromax.[29]

Ways to take azithromycin

The vast majority begin feeling much improved inside a couple of long periods of starting treatment. On the off chance that your side effects don't work on in the wake of taking azithromycin for 3-5 days or on the other hand assuming you begin feeling more awful whenever, contact your PCP.

Utilize the accompanying tips to assist with guaranteeing ideal outcomes:

Take your prescription precisely as taught.

Set a clock to diminish the gamble of failing to remember a portion.

Try not to drive or working weighty gear in the event that the drug causes you to feel tipsy.

Ask your PCP or drug specialist prior to beginning any new prescriptions or utilizing non-prescription meds or enhancements.

Azithromycin tablets can be taken regardless of food.

Azithromycin broadened discharge suspension ought to be required one hour prior or two hours in the wake of eating.

Contact your prescriber assuming you experience disturbing aftereffects.

Secondary effects causing extreme (24-hour) spewing or looseness of the bowels can slow down a few oral contraceptives.

Keep your medicine far away from youngsters and away from pets.

Azithromycin prophylaxis might be gainful for a little subgroup of patients who have rehashed intensifications of COPD, bronchiectasis or asthma. As well as antimicrobial impacts, macrolides have immunomodulatory properties and thus play a part in the administration of patients with specific provocative respiratory circumstances.

Azithromycin prophylaxis has been displayed to diminish the quantity of intensifications in patients with COPD, asthma and bronchiectasis. Thought should be given to the gamble of unfriendly impacts (gastrointestinal steamed, hearing and equilibrium aggravation, liver and cardiovascular impacts) and the improvement of antimicrobial obstruction with long haul utilization of azithromycin. The utilization of azithromycin thusly addresses an off-mark utilization of this medication however is suggested in numerous rules.

Made in the USA
Middletown, DE
01 January 2024

47051057R00035